NCCN Guidelines for Patients®

The essential guide for people facing cancer.

Based on care recommendations from leading cancer experts.

Explains high-quality cancer care provided at state-of-the-art cancer centers.

Reviewed and revised every year.

Did you know that top cancer centers across the United States work together to improve cancer care? This alliance of leading cancer centers is called the National Comprehensive Cancer Network® (NCCN®).

Because cancer care is always evolving, NCCN develops and frequently updates evidence-based cancer care recommendations used by health care providers worldwide. These recommendations are known as the NCCN Clinical Practice Guidelines in Oncology (NCCN Guidelines®).

The NCCN Guidelines for Patients plainly explain these expert recommendations, so you can talk with your care team about the best care for you.

These NCCN Guidelines for Patients are based on the NCCN Guidelines® for Myelodysplastic Syndromes, Version 3.2026 — January 12, 2026.

View the NCCN Guidelines for Patients free online: NCCN.org/patientguidelines

Find an NCCN Cancer Center near you: NCCN.org/cancercenters

Learn how the NCCN Guidelines for Patients are developed: NCCN.org/patient-guidelines-process

Connect with us

@NCCNorg @NCCNVideo NCCN @NCCNorg

Supporters

NATIONAL COMPREHENSIVE CANCER NETWORK®
NCCN FOUNDATION
Guiding Treatment. Changing Lives.

NCCN Guidelines for Patients are supported by funding from the NCCN Foundation®

NCCN Foundation gratefully acknowledges the following corporate supporters for helping to make available these NCCN Guidelines for Patients: Geron and Taiho Oncology, Inc.

NCCN independently adapts, updates, and hosts the NCCN Guidelines for Patients. Our corporate supporters do not participate in the development of the NCCN Guidelines for Patients and are not responsible for the content and recommendations contained therein.

To make a gift, visit
NCCNFoundation.org/Donate

To learn more, visit online
NCCN.org/patientguidelines
or email
PatientGuidelines@NCCN.org

Contents

NCCN Foundation seeks to support the millions of patients and their families affected by a cancer diagnosis by funding and distributing NCCN Guidelines for Patients. NCCN Foundation is also committed to advancing cancer treatment by funding the nation's promising doctors at the center of innovation in cancer research. For more details and the full library of patient and caregiver resources, visit NCCN.org/patients.

National Comprehensive Cancer Network (NCCN) and NCCN Foundation
3025 Chemical Road, Suite 100, Plymouth Meeting, PA 19462 USA

1 About MDS

Myelodysplastic syndromes (MDS) are a group of uncommon blood cancers where your bone marrow stops making enough healthy, mature blood cells. This chapter explains what MDS is and gives a brief overview of the treatments detailed later in this guide.

What is MDS?

Myelodysplastic syndromes (MDS) are a group of uncommon blood cancers.

- **myelo** means bone marrow
- **dysplastic** means growing abnormally

MDS affects your bone marrow (the soft, spongy tissue inside your bones where blood cells are made). In people with MDS, the immature blood cells in the bone marrow don't mature right. This is important because bone marrow makes many different types of blood cells, including red blood cells, white blood cells, and platelets.

Since the bone marrow isn't making normal blood cells correctly, people with MDS have low counts of 1 or more types of blood cells. It's called a **cytopenia** when you have low counts of certain types of blood cells.

What are cytopenias?

If you have a cytopenia, that means you have low counts of a certain type of blood cell. There are 3 common types of cytopenias:

1. **Anemia:** low red blood cell counts
2. **Leukopenia:** low white blood cell counts
    - **Neutropenia:** a type of leukopenia where the counts of a type of white blood cell called neutrophils are low. Neutrophils are important for fighting infections.
3. **Thrombocytopenia:** low platelet counts

What are the symptoms of MDS?

Some people with MDS don't have any **symptoms** (usually unpleasant feelings caused by a health condition), while other people do. Low blood cell counts can cause certain symptoms. The most common symptom of anemia (low red blood cell counts) is fatigue (extreme tiredness). Other common symptoms of low blood cell counts are:

- Shortness of breath (due to anemia)
- Infections or fevers that occur often (due to low counts of certain white blood cells)
- Bruising or bleeding (due to low platelet counts)

- Pale skin (due to anemia)
- Loss of appetite or weight

Sometimes symptoms can be so mild they go unnoticed too.

How is MDS found and treated?

MDS is **diagnosed** (confirmed) using blood tests and bone marrow tests, and treatment is personalized. When it's time for treatment, your care team will consider the genetic abnormalities of the MDS; whether it's lower risk or higher risk; and other factors, such as blood counts.

Treatments for MDS include:

- Different kinds of drug therapies (see *Chapter 4: Types of treatment*)
- Clinical trials (a type of medical research study that looks at new ways to fight cancer)
- Supportive care (help and services to improve your quality of life)
- A hematopoietic cell transplant (also known as a stem cell or bone marrow transplant).

There are 2 main treatment paths for MDS:

For lower-risk MDS

The main goal of treatment is **symptom management**. Your care team will focus on improving your blood cell counts and reducing the need for transfusions.

For higher-risk MDS

The main goal of treatment is **modifying the cancer**. Your care team will use stronger treatments to slow the cancer's growth. In some cases, treatment with a hematopoietic cell transplant can cure the cancer.

Will I need blood transfusions?

Most people with MDS will need a blood or platelet transfusion. Some people need many of them. Transfusions are when you receive healthy blood cells or platelets from a donor to quickly boost your counts. Getting blood or platelet transfusions can help increase low counts and can also help manage the side effects of low counts.

Can MDS change into another cancer?

Your care team will check your blood cell counts often to monitor the MDS because sometimes MDS can change into another cancer called acute myeloid leukemia (AML).

One of the goals of treatment for MDS is to reduce the risk that MDS will progress to AML.

Treatments for AML are different than those for MDS, and AML can grow quickly. For more information on AML, see *NCCN Guidelines for Patients: Acute Myeloid Leukemia*, available at NCCN.org/patientguidelines and on the NCCN Patient Guides for Cancer app.

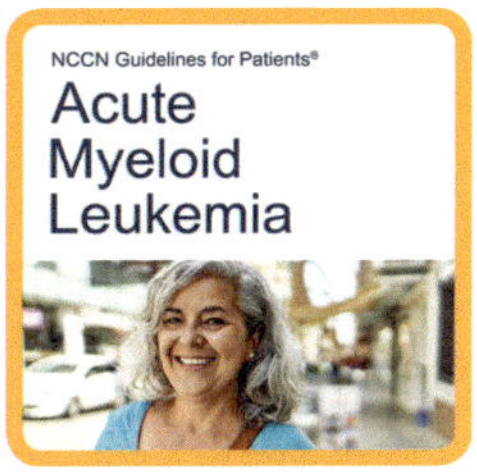

MDS affects blood stem cells made inside the bone marrow

Bone marrow contains blood stem cells (also called hematopoietic stem cells). A blood stem cell is an immature cell that can develop into blood cells, such as red blood cells, white blood cells, and platelets.

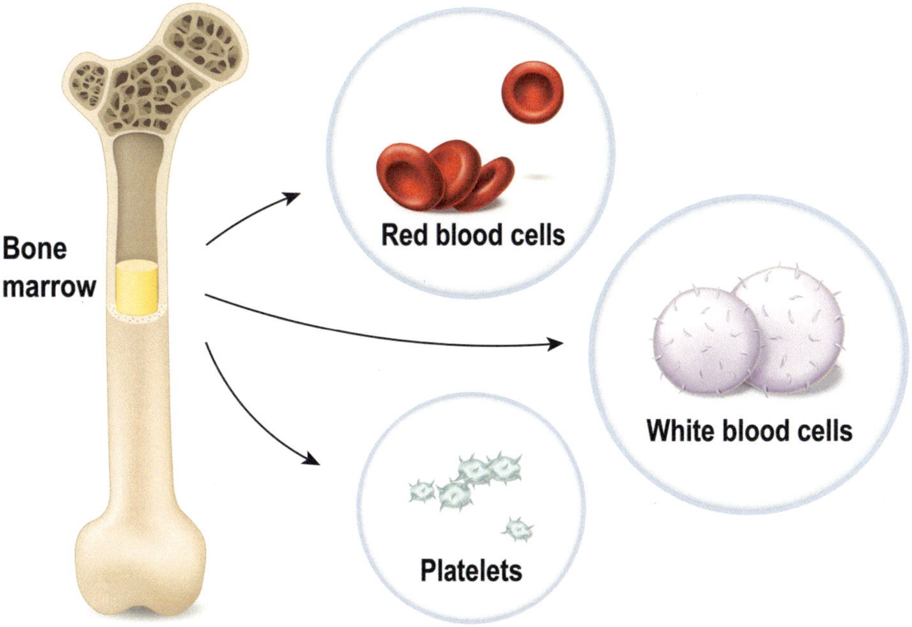

How can I get the best care?

Advocate for yourself. You have an important role to play in your care. Many people feel more satisfied when they actively take part in planning their cancer care.

The NCCN Guidelines for Patients will help you play a larger role in your care. Discuss the recommendations in this guide with your care team. Ask questions about your options and share your goals and concerns.

Don't know what to ask? You're not alone. That's why we include suggested questions to ask at the end of chapters.

Keep reading to find the best care for you.

How this guide can help you

Making decisions about cancer care is stressful. There's a lot to learn, and you don't know what the future holds.

Use this guide to get the information and support you need.

Patients, doctors, and other health care professionals trust the NCCN Guidelines for Patients. This guide uses clear, everyday language to explain current cancer care recommendations made by respected experts in the field. Their recommendations are based on the latest research and practices at leading cancer centers.

Your health is unique to you, so your cancer care should be, too. As you read this guide, you'll learn which treatments are likely to provide the best results for you. And you'll be better prepared to talk with your care team

2
Testing for MDS

Blood tests as well as a bone marrow aspiration and biopsy are used to diagnose (confirm) myelodysplastic syndromes (MDS). This chapter presents an overview of all the required tests and other tests that might be given to diagnose and plan treatment for MDS.

When will I get testing done?

Doctors or health care providers will recommend you get testing if you have cytopenias (low counts of certain types of blood cells) and if they think you might have myelodysplastic syndromes (MDS). Some tests will take a sample of your blood or bone marrow. Others may involve checking your body for signs of disease. These tests are used to figure out if you have MDS (also known as diagnosing MDS or making a diagnosis).

Medical history

Your care team needs to have all of your health information. They'll ask about any symptoms, health problems, and treatments you've had. A complete report of your health is called a **medical history**.

Diagnosis vs. prognosis

What's the difference between diagnosis and prognosis? These 2 words sound alike but they're very different.

Diagnosis: The identification of an illness based on tests. The diagnosis names what illness you have.

Prognosis: The likely course and outcome of a disease. The prognosis predicts how your disease will turn out.

When you meet with the care team, be ready to talk about your:

- Symptoms
- Illnesses
- Surgeries
- Injuries
- Health conditions
- Medications and supplements

If you've had any blood transfusions, it's also important to bring the information you have about them to your appointment. Your care team will need to see the paperwork explaining the transfusions you've had.

Family history

Some cancers and other diseases can run in families. Your care team will ask about the health history of family members who are blood relatives. This information is called a **family history**. If any family member has had cancer, it's important to know the specific type of cancer, where it started, and if it's in multiple locations.

Before you see your health care provider, you might want to ask your biological family members about their health issues and at what age they were diagnosed with them.

If you're under 50 years of age, your care team may also consider doing a genetic familial high-risk assessment. This means they'll look to see if you have any inherited genetic disorders that increase your risk of developing a bone marrow disease, such as MDS.

Physical exam

A physical exam is done to look for signs of cancer. During this exam, your doctor or health care professional may:

- Check your temperature, blood pressure, pulse, and breathing rate
- Check your height and weight
- Listen to your lungs and heart
- Look at your face and skin
- Feel and apply pressure to parts of your body to see if organs are a normal size

A list of the tests given for MDS can be found in **Guide 1**. These tests are explained in this chapter, too.

Be ready to tell your doctor about your medical history, including any family history of cancer.

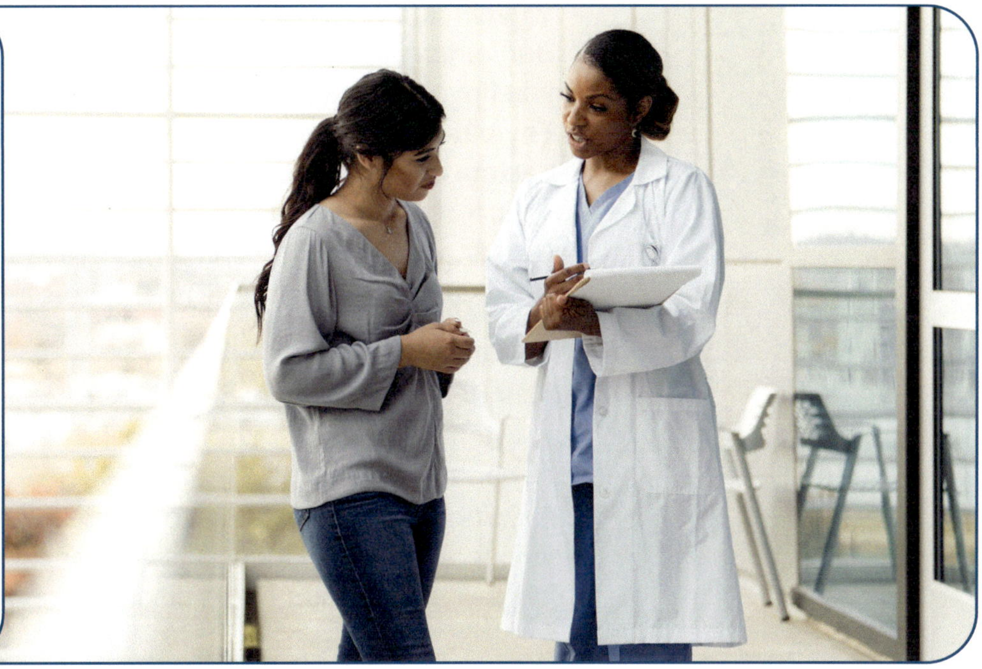

Blood tests

Blood tests are done to look for signs of cancer, and they can also show how your organs are working. A blood draw is done by inserting a needle into a vein to remove some of your blood. The blood sample is then sent to a lab for testing. At the lab, a pathologist (an expert in using lab tests to diagnose diseases) will examine the blood sample.

The blood sample may be used for the following tests:

Complete blood count with differential

A complete blood count measures the levels of red blood cells, white blood cells, and platelets in your blood. A differential counts the number of each type of white blood cell. It can also show if there are immature white blood cells (called blasts) in the blood. Cancer and other health problems can cause low or high blood cell counts.

Guide 1
Tests and procedures for MDS

Needed or recommended	• Medical history and physical exam • Bone marrow aspiration and biopsy • Blood tests: - Complete blood count with differential, platelet, and reticulocyte count - Blood smear examination - Serum erythropoietin (EPO) levels (before a red blood cell transfusion is given) - Vitamin B12 and folate levels - Serum ferritin, iron, total iron-binding capacity (TIBC) test (to see if you have too much or not enough iron) - Thyroid-stimulating hormone (TSH) levels - Lactate dehydrogenase (LDH) levels • Genetic testing for certain mutations • Molecular and genetic testing for inherited genetic disorders (mainly for people under 50 years of age)
Needed in some cases	• HIV testing • Copper deficiency evaluation • Flow cytometry to help with diagnosis • More genetic testing • HLA typing (if you might receive a transplant) • Testing to see if the diagnosis is congenital sideroblastic anemia (CSA), which is an uncommon blood disorder, not MDS

Reticulocyte count

Reticulocytes are young red blood cells in your bone marrow. A reticulocyte count can help your care team find out if your bone marrow is producing enough healthy red blood cells. If you have anemia, a reticulocyte count can also help your health care provider find the cause of the anemia.

Blood smear

A blood smear examines a sample of your blood by looking at the size, shape, and number of blood cells. It may also be used to see if there are blast cells in the bloodstream.

Blood tests are used to help diagnose and plan treatment for MDS.

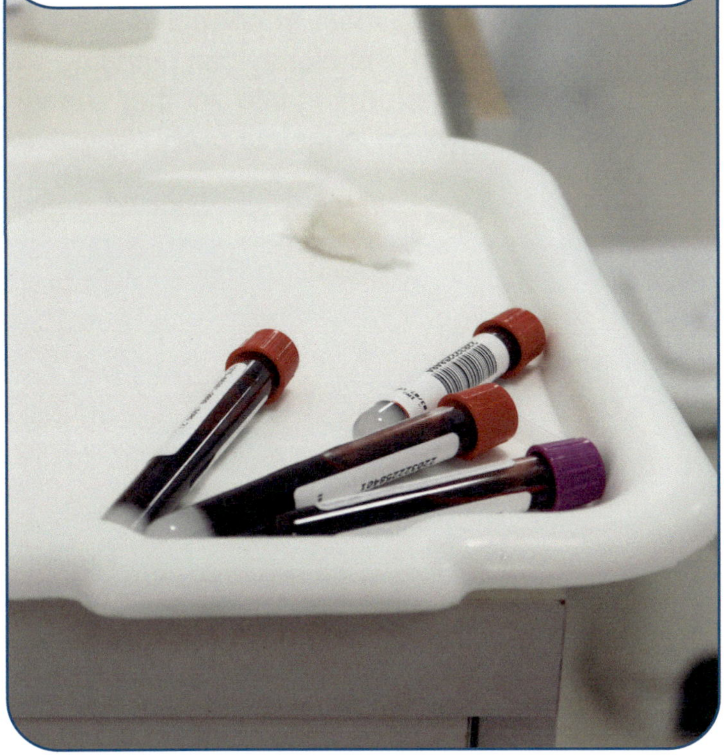

Serum erythropoietin levels

Erythropoietin (also called EPO) is a hormone your kidneys produce that causes the bone marrow to make red blood cells. If you have anemia, measuring the amount of erythropoietin in your blood can also help your health care provider figure out what type of anemia you have. Most people with anemia that's caused by MDS have erythropoietin levels that are higher than normal.

Vitamin B12 and folate levels

Measuring the levels of vitamin B12 and folate in your blood is important to see if the levels are within a normal range. Lower levels of vitamin B12 or folate can cause anemia and other issues, such as fatigue (feeling tired).

Iron and ferritin levels

Your body needs iron to function properly. A total iron-binding capacity (also called TIBC) test will be done to measure the protein that carries iron in your blood. If you don't have enough iron in your body, the TIBC is usually elevated, but in MDS the TIBC is expected to be normal.

Testing levels of ferritin (a protein that stores iron) is also important. You will have a ferritin test to help your care team understand how much iron is being stored in your body. If your ferritin levels are lower than normal, your body doesn't have enough iron. Low levels of iron can cause anemia.

Thyroid-stimulating hormone levels

Your thyroid (a gland in the neck) makes hormones that control how your body uses energy. A thyroid-stimulating hormone (also called TSH) test measures levels of the hormone to learn more about your health. Occasionally, severely low thyroid function can cause anemia.

Lactate dehydrogenase levels

Lactate dehydrogenase (LDH) is a protein found in almost all cells. When cells die, they release LDH into the blood. High levels of LDH can be caused by cancer or other health problems. LDH tests are done for many different reasons, including to see how serious certain cancers are. However, the role of LDH testing in MDS is limited.

Bone marrow tests

MDS is a cancer of the bone marrow (the spongy tissue in the center of most bones where blood cells are made). To diagnose MDS and figure out what type of MDS you have, samples of bone marrow must be taken and tested.

A bone marrow aspiration and biopsy are 2 types of bone marrow tests that are often done at the same time. Bone marrow aspiration removes liquid bone marrow. Bone marrow biopsy removes bone marrow tissue. Both samples are usually taken from the back of the hip bone. In certain situations, the bone marrow aspiration sample may be taken from the sternal bone (breast bone). After your health care provider gets the samples, they'll be sent to a lab for testing.

A bone marrow aspiration and biopsy might be done again after treatment to see how the MDS is responding to treatment. Also, if blood cell counts become more abnormal, a bone marrow aspiration and biopsy can help find out if MDS is transforming into another cancer called acute myeloid leukemia (AML).

Understanding the bone marrow aspiration and biopsy procedure

A bone marrow aspiration and biopsy usually takes about 15 minutes. Here's what to expect:

Step 1: Getting Ready
First, you'll lie on your side or stomach, depending on where the sample will be taken (it's usually taken from your hip bone). The area will be cleaned, you may be given medication to help you relax, and your vital signs will be checked.

2

Step 2: Numbing the Area
Next, the doctor will numb the area with an injection. Then the doctor will make a very small cut in your skin.

Step 3: Taking the Samples
The doctor will collect 2 samples through the cut. You'll need to stay very still during these few minutes.

First, the aspiration: A needle goes into the bone to remove liquid bone marrow. You may feel pressure or a pulling sensation that lasts a few seconds.

Then, the biopsy: A special needle twists gently into the bone to remove a small piece of solid bone marrow tissue. You might feel some pressure or a dull ache.

4

Step 4: Finishing Up
Once the samples are collected, the doctor will put a bandage on the area and you'll rest for about 15 minutes to make sure there's no bleeding. Most people can return to normal activities the same day, but you might feel sore or stiff.

Genetic tests

MDS treatment can sometimes be based on the genetic abnormalities of the MDS and whether it's lower risk or higher risk. So genetic testing is important. Genetic testing looks for changes in genes and chromosomes known to be related to MDS. Your care team may also ask about your personal and family history of cancer, since some genetic changes are hereditary (passed down from biological parents to children). People under 50 years of age will likely have additional genetic testing and molecular testing done.

To look for chromosome and genetic changes (abnormalities) in the cancer cells, your care team will use cytogenetic testing and molecular testing. Cytogenetic testing examines chromosomes and includes the fluorescence in situ hybridization (FISH) test and a karyotype. Molecular testing examines the genes (segments of DNA) and includes polymerase chain reaction (PCR) testing and next-generation sequencing (NGS). These tests are explained next.

Cytogenetic testing

Cytogenetic testing uses samples of tissue, blood, or bone marrow to look for changes and abnormalities in chromosomes. There are many types of chromosome abnormalities. Part of a chromosome may be missing, a whole chromosome may be missing, or there may be an extra copy of a chromosome.

Identifying the type and number of chromosome changes can help your care team choose a treatment for you. Some treatments work better for MDS with certain chromosome changes than other treatments do.

Health care providers use symbols and shortened terms to describe the different types of chromosome changes. A missing chromosome or missing part of a chromosome is noted by a minus sign (–) or the word del, for deletion. An extra copy of a chromosome is noted by a plus sign (+).

Examples of chromosome abnormalities in MDS include:

- del(5q), or 5q deletion, which means part of the "q," or longer part of chromosome 5, is missing
- del(7), which means part of chromosome 7 is missing

About half of people with MDS have at least 1 chromosome change. The most common abnormalities are found on chromosomes 5, 7, 8, and 20.

FISH testing detects specific common chromosome changes known to affect people with MDS. The test is done on samples of your blood, tissue, or bone marrow. FISH testing looks into a very specific part of a certain chromosome and doesn't show all chromosomes.

A **karyotype** is a picture of all of someone's chromosomes. It's made with a sample of your blood or body fluid. Karyotypes are used to look for any abnormal changes in the chromosomes and any abnormalities with the number of chromosomes.

Molecular testing

A **PCR test** creates more copies of a specific gene so your DNA can be better examined. This test can find genetic changes and is done using a sample of body fluid.

NGS checks the sequence (order) of your genes to look for mutations and changes. It also looks at the genes in a more detailed way than other testing methods and can find mutations other methods might miss. The test uses a sample of your blood or tissue.

Flow cytometry

Flow cytometry is a lab test used to help diagnose MDS. It's a laser based test that uses a blood, tissue, or bone marrow sample to count, identify, sort, and classify cells.

Additional tests that might be done

Sometimes more genetic tests or other types of tests are needed to diagnose and plan treatment for people with MDS. The other tests you might get are described below.

Copper level examination

Your care team may recommend a copper level test because low levels can cause a low neutrophil count and/or anemia. The test is done to make sure the anemia or low neutrophil count isn't being caused by a copper deficiency.

HIV testing

If needed, your care team may also test you for HIV. HIV can cause low blood cell counts and anemia, so in certain cases tests may be done to make sure HIV isn't causing the low blood cell count.

Testing if you might get a transplant: HLA typing

Sometimes people with MDS are treated with a hematopoietic cell transplant (also called a bone marrow or stem cell transplant) to kick-start the bone marrow into making healthy blood cells. An allogeneic hemopoietic cell transplant is a type of transplant that replaces the unhealthy stem cells in your bone marrow with healthy donated stem cells.

If your care team thinks you may need a hemopoietic cell transplant, they will do a blood test called human leukocyte antigen (HLA) typing. This test helps find a donor whose stem cells are the best match for you. HLA is different in different people, and a donor has to have an HLA that is close to your HLA. Finding a donor isn't based on blood type, it's based on the HLA type.

Key points

- Blood tests and a bone marrow aspiration and biopsy are used to diagnose myelodysplastic syndromes (MDS).
- Many different tests are done on your blood to learn more about the MDS and low blood cell counts.
- A medical history, physical exam, and flow cytometry will also be done and can reveal signs of cancer.
- It's important to bring information about any transfusions you've had with you when you meet with your care team.
- Genetic testing is very important because treatment for MDS is based on the genetic abnormalities of the MDS and whether it's lower risk or higher risk. Genetic tests check for abnormal changes in the genes and chromosomes of MDS cells.

Questions to ask

- Will I get all my testing done at the same place?
- What assistance is available to help me pay for testing or transportation to my appointments?
- How long will it take to get my test results back?
- Who will explain the test results to me and when?
- How often will I need to have blood tests done?

3
Types of MDS

There are many types of myelodysplastic syndromes (MDS), and treatment depends on several different factors. This chapter explains the types of MDS, risk groups for MDS, and how your care team will pick treatments for you.

The types of MDS

To figure out what type of myelodysplastic syndromes (MDS) you have, your care team will look at the genetic and chromosome abnormalities (also called mutations, or changes), features of your bone marrow and blood cells, and how many blasts (immature blood cells) are in your bone marrow.

As doctors, researchers, and care teams learn more about MDS, the names for the types of MDS have been changing. The most recent publication from the World Health Organization (WHO) on how to describe and classify the types of MDS was published in 2022. A list of the types of MDS per the WHO can be found in **Guide 2**.

Additionally, although it's uncommon, sometimes blood cancer can have features of MDS and a different bone marrow disease called myeloproliferative neoplasms (MPN). MDS/MPN overlap syndromes are when the cancer has characteristics of both MDS and MPN. *Chapter 7: MDS/MPN overlap syndromes* explains these syndromes and how they're treated.

Lower-risk MDS includes people with a very low, low, or intermediate risk of disease.

Higher-risk MDS includes people with an intermediate, high, or very high risk of disease.

Risk groups

Care teams and doctors will treat MDS based on whether it's lower risk or higher risk. Your care team will use a risk scoring system to figure out the MDS risk group. There are a few different scoring systems that can be used, but NCCN and most treatment providers use the Revised International Prognostic Scoring System (IPSS-R). This scoring system sorts MDS into the following 5 groups:

- Very low risk
- Low risk
- Intermediate risk
- High risk
- Very high risk

These 5 MDS groups can be sorted into 2 basic risk categories: **lower risk** and **higher risk**. NCCN experts make treatment recommendations based on if the MDS is lower or higher risk. Your care team may also use a more precise risk classification method called the International Prognostic Scoring System Molecular (IPSS-M) to help figure out the outcome of the cancer (prognosis). IPSS-M

Guide 2
Types of MDS

MDS with low blasts (MDS-LB)	There are a low number of immature blood cells (blasts) in the blood and bone marrow.
MDS with 5q deletion (MDS-5q)	Cells have a change known as the 5q deletion, which means that part of chromosome 5 is missing (deleted).
MDS with *SF3B1* mutation (MDS-*SF3B1*)	Cells have a mutation in the *SF3B1* gene.
MDS, hypoplastic (MDS-h)	There are fewer cells in the bone marrow than usual.
MDS with biallelic *TP53* inactivation (MDS-bi*TP53*)	There is a genetic abnormality where the TP53 protein is not active.
MDS with increased blasts (MDS-IB)	There are a greater number of blasts in the blood and bone marrow. Sometimes, this type of MDS is further defined as MDS-IB1 and MDS-IB2 to describe the number of blasts. MDS-IB2 has a higher number of blasts than MDS-IB1.
MDS with fibrosis (MDS-f)	Scar-like tissue (fibrosis) has built up in the bone marrow.
Acute myeloid leukemia (AML)	For about 1 in 3 people with MDS, MDS changes into another cancer called AML. For more information on AML, see *NCCN Guidelines for Patients: Acute Myeloid Leukemia.*

builds on the IPSS-R scoring system by adding information about specific mutations to its scoring system.

To figure out the cancer's risk group, the scoring system looks at certain factors related to the genetic profile of the MDS, your blood counts, and your bone marrow. Other factors include:

- The number of blast cells in the bone marrow
- How low some of the blood cell counts (cytopenias) are
- The type and number of chromosome changes (cytogenetic changes)

How will my care team pick treatments?

Treatment for MDS is personalized and depends on many different factors. To make a treatment plan, your care team will first see if you have lower-risk or higher-risk MDS.

The treatment you receive also depends on other factors, such as:

- If you have symptomatic anemia
- If the cancer has genetic abnormalities, such as a 5q deletion (known as having the MDS-5q subtype) or a *SF3B1* mutation (known as having the MDS-*SF3B1* subtype)
- What your serum erythropoietin (EPO) level is (EPO is a hormone that triggers your bone marrow to make red blood cells)
- If the cancer has an *IDH1* or *IDH2* mutation
- If you're able to receive a hematopoietic cell transplant

Who's on your care team?

Treating MDS takes a team approach. Some members of your care team will be with you throughout treatment, while others will be there for parts of it. Your team should communicate and work together to bring the best knowledge from each specialty together.

Your care team may include:

- medical oncologists and hematologists
- nurses
- pharmacists
- physician assistants
- patient navigators
- social workers
- nutritionists
- other specialists

Key points

- There are many different types of myelodysplastic syndromes (MDS). To find out what type of MDS you have, your care team will look at the genetic abnormalities found, features of your bone marrow and blood cells, and how many blasts (immature cells) are in your blood.
- Care teams and doctors treat MDS based on whether it's lower risk or higher risk. Other factors are considered, too.
- Lower-risk MDS includes people with very low-risk, low-risk, and intermediate-risk disease.
- Higher-risk MDS includes people with intermediate-risk, high-risk, and very high-risk disease.
- The treatment you receive also depends on factors such as what genetic or chromosome abnormalities you have, the number of blasts in your bone marrow, what your serum erythropoietin (EPO) level is, and if you're able to receive a hematopoietic cell transplant.

Questions to ask

- Is the MDS lower risk or higher risk? What does it mean to have intermediate-risk MDS? Can you tell me more about risk status?
- What treatment options are available for my type of MDS?
- Is there a hospital or doctor near me that specializes in MDS treatment? Can I get a second opinion there before treatment starts?
- Who is on my care team, and which person can help me find resources to help pay for treatment?
- How long should I wait after testing to start treatment? What if I don't start treatment right away?

What's next?

Now that your care team knows what type of MDS you have and what risk group the MDS is in, they can start planning treatment. The next chapter describes the different types of available treatments. It also explains what supportive care is and how it can help you.

4
Types of treatment

Many treatments are available for myelodysplastic syndromes (MDS). Your care team will work with you to find the best treatment option for the type of MDS you have. This chapter talks about the different types of treatment and specific drug options. There's also information about clinical trials and supportive care.

There are several different types of treatments that can be given for myelodysplastic syndromes (MDS). **Guide 3** lists the types of treatments, and they're described in more detail below. *Chapter 5: Treating lower-risk MDS* and *Chapter 6: Treating higher-risk MDS* explain when different treatments are recommended and if they are preferred therapies, other recommended therapies, or therapies used in certain cases.

Guide 3 Types of treatments for MDS
Chemotherapy and hypomethylating agents
Targeted therapy
Therapies involving the immune system • Immunomodulating drugs • Immunosuppressive therapy
Erythropoiesis-stimulating agents (also called ESAs)
Erythroid maturation agents (also called EMAs)
Granulocyte colony-stimulating factors (also called G-CSFs)
Thrombopoietin receptor agonists
Hematopoietic cell transplant (also called a bone marrow or stem cell transplant)
Clinical trials

What is systemic therapy?

Systemic therapy is treatment that works throughout the entire body. These therapies travel through the bloodstream to destroy cancer cells all over the body. Chemotherapy and targeted therapy are types of systemic therapy.

All treatments listed in this guide are recommended and appropriate. When helpful, NCCN experts also assign a level of preference to their recommendations for systemic therapies:

- **Preferred therapies** have the most evidence they may work better and be safer than other therapies.
- **Other recommended therapies** can provide effective results but may have less evidence, more side effects, or may not work quite as well as preferred therapies.
- **Therapies used in certain cases** work best for individuals with specific cancer features or health circumstances.

Chemotherapy and hypomethylating agents

Chemotherapy drugs kill cancer cells throughout the body. Different types of chemotherapy drugs work in different ways to kill cancer cells or stop new ones from being made. In certain cases, high-intensity chemotherapy can be used, but hypomethylating agents are standard therapy for treating MDS. **Hypomethylating agents are sometimes called chemotherapy since they're given through a vein like chemotherapy, but they are their own type of drug.**

The 3 hypomethylating agents commonly given to treat MDS are:

- Azacitidine (Vidaza)
  - Given as an injection under your skin (subcutaneous injection) or injected slowly into a vein (IV infusion)
- Decitabine
  - Given as an IV infusion
- Decitabine and cedazuridine (Inqovi)
  - Given as tablets you can take

Targeted therapies

Targeted therapy is a type of treatment that targets specific features of cancer cells. There are many different types of targeted therapy, and these are the ones that are used to treat MDS:

Imetelstat (Rytelo)

Imetelstat is a type of targeted therapy called a telomerase inhibitor that's given as an IV infusion. People with lower-risk MDS and anemia are often treated with this drug.

Ivosidenib (Tibsovo)

Ivosidenib is a tablet that's given as a treatment for people who have an *IDH1* mutation. IDH1 is a gene that can be mutated (changed) in MDS. Ivosidenib is a type of targeted therapy called an IDH1 inhibitor.

Enasidenib (Idhifa)

Enasidenib is a tablet that's used to treat people with MDS who have an *IDH2* mutation. IDH2 is a gene that can be mutated in MDS, and enasidenib is a type of targeted therapy called an IDH2 inhibitor.

Venetoclax (Venclexta)

Venetoclax is a type of targeted therapy called a BCL-2 inhibitor that's given as tablets. Certain people with higher-risk MDS may receive venetoclax in combination with a hypomethylating agent.

Erythropoiesis-stimulating agents

Erythropoiesis-stimulating agents (also called ESAs) are drugs that kick-start the bone marrow to make more red blood cells. People who have lower-risk MDS with anemia may receive an ESA as part of their treatment. The 2 available ESAs are:

- Epoetin alfa (Epogen and Procrit)
- Darbepoetin alfa (Aranesp)

These are both given as an injection under your skin.

Erythroid maturation agent

Luspatercept-aamt (Reblozyl) is an erythroid maturation agent (also called EMA) that's given as an injection under the skin. It's used to treat people with lower-risk MDS who have anemia.

Immunomodulatory drug

People with lower-risk MDS and anemia sometimes receive the immunomodulatory drug lenalidomide (Revlimid) during treatment. It's given as a capsule.

Granulocyte colony-stimulating factor

Sometimes, a type of drug called a granulocyte colony-stimulating factor (G-CSF) can be combined with other treatments or given by itself for people with lower-risk MDS. These drugs help increase the number of white blood cells, and white blood cells are important to help your body fight infections. Filgrastim (Neupogen) is a G-CSF that you might receive. It's given as an injection under your skin.

Immunosuppressive therapies

Immunosuppressive therapy (also called IST) lowers the activity of your immune system. Some people with lower-risk MDS can receive this therapy to prevent the immune system from attacking healthy cells (such as the healthy bone marrow cells that make blood cells). The immunosuppressive therapies you might get for MDS are:

- Anti-thymocyte globulin, also called ATG (Atgam), which is given as an IV infusion
- Cyclosporine A (Sandimmune and Neoral), which is given orally for MDS (as an oral solution or capsules)

ATG and cyclosporine A are given together, and sometimes the drug eltrombopag is given with them.

Thrombopoietin receptor agonists

Eltrombopag (Promacta and Alvaiz) is a type of drug called a thrombopoietin receptor agonist that's given as tablets. It's given in combination with immunosuppressive therapy. People with lower-risk MDS, particularly with low platelet counts, can receive this drug in certain situations.

Romiplostim (Nplate) is another thrombopoietin receptor agonist. It's used to treat people with MDS who have low platelet counts and it's given as an injection under your skin.

Allogeneic hematopoietic cell transplant

If you get a hematopoietic cell transplant, the type you will receive is called an **allogeneic hematopoietic cell transplant**. An allogeneic transplant uses healthy stem cells from another person (donor) to regrow your bone marrow. First, you'll receive treatment with chemotherapy and/or radiation therapy to kill the cancer cells in the bone marrow. Next, you'll receive an infusion of healthy stem cells from a donor. These cells form new, healthy bone marrow, which will make healthy blood cells.

Before the transplant, special testing must be done to make sure the donor is a match for you. Human leukocyte antigen (HLA) typing is used to figure out which donor is the best match for you.

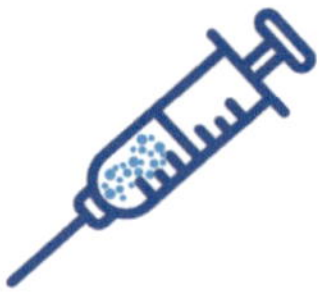

Hematopoietic cell transplant

A hematopoietic cell transplant may also be called called a bone marrow transplant or stem cell transplant. It's a type of treatment that replaces blood-producing (hematopoietic) stem cells that have been destroyed by high doses of chemotherapy. An allogeneic hematopoietic cell transplant is the type of transplant that's given for MDS. It uses healthy stem cells from another person (donor) to regrow your bone marrow.

A hematopoietic cell transplant is an intense treatment and isn't for everyone. Talk to your care team to see if it might be a good fit for you or if other therapy would be better.

Clinical trials

A clinical trial is a type of medical research study. After being developed and tested in a lab, potential new ways of fighting cancer need to be studied in people.

If found to be safe and effective in a clinical trial, a drug, device, or treatment approach may be approved by the U.S. FDA.

Everyone with cancer should carefully consider all of the treatment options available for their cancer type, including standard treatments and clinical trials. Talk to your doctor about whether a clinical trial may make sense for you.

Phases

Most cancer clinical trials focus on treatment and are done in phases.

- **Phase 1** trials study the safety and side effects of an investigational drug or treatment approach.
- **Phase 2** trials study how well the drug or approach works against a specific type of cancer.
- **Phase 3** trials test the drug or approach against a standard treatment. If the results are good, it may be approved by the FDA.
- **Phase 4** trials study the safety and benefit of an FDA-approved treatment.

Who can enroll?

It depends on the clinical trial's rules, called eligibility criteria. The rules may be about age, cancer type and stage, treatment history, or general health. They ensure that participants are alike in specific ways and that the trial is as safe as possible for the participants.

Informed consent

Clinical trials are managed by a research team. This group of experts will review the study with you in detail, including its purpose and the risks and benefits of joining. All of this information is also provided in an informed consent form. Read the form carefully and

Finding a clinical trial

In the United States

NCCN Cancer Centers
NCCN.org/cancercenters

The National Cancer Institute (NCI)
cancer.gov/about-cancer/treatment/clinical-trials/search

Worldwide

The U.S. National Library of Medicine (NLM)
clinicaltrials.gov

Need help finding a clinical trial?

NCI's Cancer Information Service (CIS)
1.800.4.CANCER (1.800.422.6237)
cancer.gov/contact

ask questions before signing it. Take time to discuss it with people you trust. Keep in mind that you can leave and seek treatment outside of the clinical trial at any time.

Will I get a placebo?

Placebos (inactive versions of real medicines) are almost never used alone in cancer clinical trials. It is common to receive either a placebo with a standard treatment, or a new drug with a standard treatment. You will be informed, verbally and in writing, if a placebo is part of a clinical trial before you enroll.

Are clinical trials free?

There is no fee to enroll in a clinical trial. The study sponsor pays for research-related costs, including the study drug. But you may need to pay for other services, like transportation or childcare, due to extra appointments. During the trial, you will continue to receive standard cancer care. This care is often covered by insurance.

Supportive care

Supportive care is an important part of cancer care. The goal is to improve your quality of life during and after cancer treatment. Supportive care is for everyone with cancer and their families, not just for those at the end of life.

Supportive care includes a wide range of services. Supportive care prevents or manages the symptoms of cancer and the side effects of cancer treatment, like pain and cancer-related fatigue (tiredness). It also addresses the mental, social, emotional, and spiritual concerns you may have.

Supportive care provides help with additional needs, such as:

- Making treatment decisions
- Coordinating your care
- Paying for care
- Planning for advance care and end of life

To read more about the types of support you may receive see *NCCN Guidelines for Patients: Palliative Care*, available at NCCN.org/patientguidelines and on the NCCN Patient Guides for Cancer app.

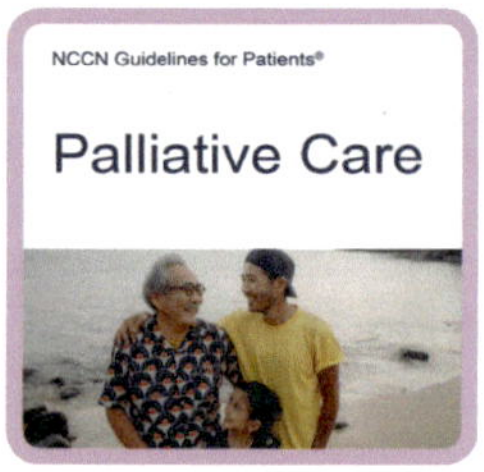

Supportive care specific to MDS

Supportive care can help improve your quality of life by reducing symptoms caused by low blood counts, including low red blood cells (anemia). Cancer treatments can also cause unwanted health issues, known as side effects. Side effects depend on many factors, such as the type of drug and dose received, how long treatment is given for, and the person.

Ask your care team for a list of your treatment's side effects, and tell them about any symptoms that are new or getting worse. There may be ways to help you feel better and prevent some side effects before they happen or get worse.

Supportive care that's given for MDS in particular includes the following:

Emotional and social support

Psychosocial support is help for emotional, mental, social, and spiritual needs. This can include counseling, education, and support groups. Distress can also be a common feeling during cancer care. *NCCN Guidelines for Patients: Distress During Cancer Care,* are available at NCCN.org/patientguidelines and on the NCCN Patient Guides for Cancer app.

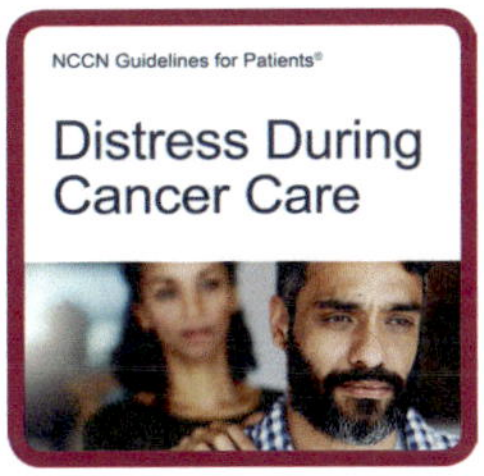

Checking on quality of life

A quality-of-life assessment is used to identify concerns, such as pain or other problems, that may be physical, social, or spiritual. This helps your care team manage any concerns or difficulties. Several questionnaires and surveys are available to help your care team evaluate your quality of life.

Transfusions and help afterward

People with MDS experiencing symptoms of anemia can benefit from a transfusion of red blood cells and treatment with erythropoiesis-stimulating agents. People with thrombocytopenia (low platelet counts) and bleeding can benefit from a platelet transfusion and certain medications. These transfusions help manage the symptoms of anemia (such as fatigue and shortness of breath) and the symptoms of thrombocytopenia (such as bruising and bleeding).

However, receiving 20 or more red blood cell transfusions might cause iron to build up in the body (iron overload) and that can cause damage to organs, such as the heart, liver, and pancreas. Iron chelation therapy is given to treat iron overload and includes deferoxamine, which is given as an injection under the skin, or deferasirox, which is given as a tablet.

If thrombocytopenia is severe or life-threatening, a thrombopoietin receptor agonist may be given to increase your platelet counts. If it's needed or if bleeding hasn't gotten better with platelet transfusions, a drug called an anti-fibrinolytic agent (such as aminocaproic acid) may be given.

Help after a transplant

If you've had a hematopoietic cell transplant and are currently being treated with immunosuppressive therapy, you'll receive medicine to help prevent infections (sometimes called antimicrobial prophylaxis). Preventive infection-fighting medicines can include antibiotics.

Antibiotics for bacterial infections

People with MDS who have a low white blood cell count can get infections. Antibiotics are usually given to treat bacterial infections.

Key points

- Systemic therapy is treatment that works throughout the entire body, such as chemotherapy and targeted therapy.
- NCCN experts assign a level of preference to their recommendations for systemic therapies. Treatments that are recommended can be preferred therapies, other recommended therapies, or therapies used in certain cases.
- Treatments for myelodysplastic syndromes (MDS) are chemotherapy, hypomethylating agents, targeted therapies, immunosuppressive therapies, erythropoiesis-stimulating agents, erythroid maturation agents, immunomodulatory drugs, granulocyte colony-stimulating factors, thrombopoietin receptor agonists, allogeneic hematopoietic cell transplant, and clinical trials.
- An allogeneic hematopoietic cell transplant uses chemotherapy to destroy cells in the bone marrow and then replaces them with healthy, blood-forming cells from a donor.
- A clinical trial is a type of medical research study that studies potential new ways of fighting cancer in people. Ask your care team if there are any clinical trials available that are a good fit for you.
- Supportive care includes a wide range of services, and its goal is to improve your quality of life during and after cancer treatment. Supportive care is for everyone with cancer and their families.
- Supportive care for MDS can also help improve your quality of life by reducing symptoms from low blood counts, including low red blood cells (anemia).

Questions to ask

- Can you recommend a health care professional, hospital, or cancer center that specializes in MDS?
- Which treatments are recommended for me and why?
- What are the most common side effects of MDS treatments? How can supportive care help with these side effects?
- What should I do if I have side effects when the doctor's office isn't open?
- Are there resources to help pay for treatment or any other care I might need?

5
Treating lower-risk MDS

Treatment options for lower-risk myelodysplastic syndromes (MDS) vary, depending on what type of lower-risk MDS you have. This chapter describes what treatments are given for people who have lower-risk MDS with significantly low blood cell counts and different types of symptomatic anemia.

It's important to know that if you have lower-risk myelodysplastic syndromes (MDS) without symptoms, you may not need treatment right away. Instead, you'll go to regular checkups, your blood counts will be monitored, and you might receive supportive care. This is referred to as active monitoring, or "watching and waiting."

However, if you have lower-risk MDS with anemia and are having some symptoms, you may need treatment. This chapter explains the treatments that are recommended for the different types of lower-risk MDS.

Treatments for MDS with significantly low blood cell counts

If you have MDS with cytopenias (low counts of certain types of blood cells) that your care team thinks are significant, you'll receive supportive care with your main treatment. To learn more about supportive care, see *Chapter 4: Types of treatment*.

Your main treatment depends on which type of blood cell is low. If you have thrombocytopenia (low platelet counts) or neutropenia (low levels of neutrophils, a type of white blood cell), you'll receive 1 of the treatments in **Guide 4**. If you have symptomatic anemia, see the section "Treatment for MDS with symptomatic anemia" on page 35.

Examining treatment-related anemia

Before people with symptomatic anemia can be treated, it's important to learn as much about the anemia as possible. You'll receive some of the same tests and exams that you had before to check on the anemia (see *Chapter 2: Testing for MDS* for more information). These are the tests and exams that may be done again:

- Medical history and physical exam
- Blood tests including a complete blood count with differential, platelet, and reticulocyte count; serum erythropoietin (EPO) levels; and blood smear examination
- Bone marrow aspiration, biopsy, and cytogenetics

Your care team will also make sure something else isn't causing the anemia. If that's the case, they'll treat whatever the cause is. They may also give you supportive care and red blood cell transfusions, if needed.

Treatments for MDS with symptomatic anemia

If you have symptomatic anemia, the treatment you get depends on many factors, such as the genetic characteristics of the MDS. NCCN experts recommend certain treatments for people with:

1. Symptomatic anemia and the 5q deletion (MDS-5q)
   - This means the cancer has the 5q deletion, low blasts, and might have 1 other cytogenetic abnormality (except ones involving chromosome 7).
2. Symptomatic anemia and the *SF3B1* mutation (MDS-SF3B1)
   - This means the cancer has the *SF3B1* mutation, low blasts, and a certain amount of ring sideroblasts (immature red blood cells with too much iron). This type of MDS might have other cytogenetic abnormalities, too, but it doesn't have the 5q deletion.
3. Symptomatic anemia and no 5q deletion, with or without other cytogenetic abnormalities. A certain number of ring sideroblasts are also found.

Guide 4
Treatments for MDS with clinically relevant thrombocytopenia or neutropenia

First treatment	• Clinical trial • Azacitidine • Decitabine • Decitabine and cedazuridine • Immunosuppressive therapy with or without eltrombopag (useful in certain circumstances)		
If the cancer doesn't respond to treatment, progresses, or comes back after it went away (relapses), the treatments listed next will be given.			
Next treatments	• Azacitidine, decitabine, or decitabine and cedazuridine (if not given yet) • Ivosidenib, if the *IDH1* gene is mutated • Enasidenib, if the *IDH2* gene is mutated	→	• Clinical trial • Allogeneic hematopoietic cell transplant (for certain people) • Ivosidenib, if there is an *IDH1* mutation and the drug hasn't been given yet • Enasidenib, if there is an *IDH2* mutation and the drug hasn't been given yet

Lower-risk MDS includes Revised International Prognostic Scoring System (IPSS-R) very low-risk, low-risk, and intermediate-risk groups.

Treatments for lower-risk MDS with symptomatic anemia and the 5q deletion

If you have MDS with the 5q deletion, the first treatment you'll get depends on the amount of serum erythropoietin (EPO) in your blood. Erythropoietin is a hormone in the body that tells the bone marrow to make more red blood cells. The first treatment options for MDS with the 5q deletion are listed in **Guide 5**.

If the cancer is responding to treatment, then the treatment will be continued and the dose might be decreased to help with side effects. If the cancer isn't responding to treatment or relapses, then more treatments will be given.

The additional treatments for MDS with symptomatic anemia and the 5q deletion are described next on page 37.

Treatments for lower-risk MDS with symptomatic anemia and the *SF3B1* mutation

If you have MDS with symptomatic anemia and the *SF3B1* mutation, you can receive the following treatments:

- Luspatercept-aamt (Reblozyl) (preferred)
- Imetelstat (Rytelo) (other recommended), given to people with a serum EPO level greater than 500 mU/mL who can't receive epoetin alfa or darbepoetin alfa

Guide 5
First treatments for lower-risk MDS with symptomatic anemia and the 5q deletion

For people with a serum EPO level of 500 mU/mL or less:	• Lenalidomide (preferred) • Epoetin alfa (other recommended) • Darbepoetin alfa (other recommended)
For people with a serum EPO level more than 500 mU/mL:	• Lenalidomide (preferred)

Additional treatments for lower-risk MDS with symptomatic anemia and the 5q deletion

If your care team thinks immunosuppressive therapy may be a good option for you, you'll be treated with anti-thymocyte globulin (ATG) plus cyclosporine A with or without eltrombopag.

If the cancer doesn't respond to immunosuppressive therapy or if your care team doesn't think immunosuppressive therapy is the right option, then you can get the following treatments:

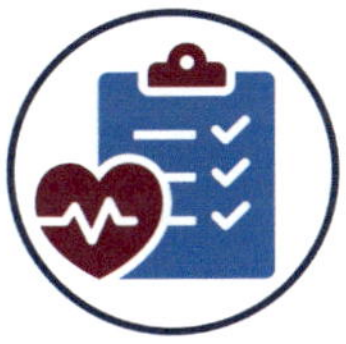

- Imetelstat, if not given yet (preferred)
- Clinical trial
- Azacitidine (other recommended)
- Decitabine (other recommended)
- Decitabine and cedazuridine (other recommended)
- Lenalidomide (useful in certain circumstances)

If the cancer doesn't respond to therapy or relapses, the following treatments can be given:

- Clinical trial
- Allogeneic hematopoietic cell transplantation (for certain people)
- Ivosidenib, if not given yet for MDS with *IDH1* mutations
- Enasidenib, if not given yet for MDS with *IDH2* mutations

If the cancer doesn't respond to treatment or relapses, then the next treatment you'll get depends on your serum EPO level. The treatment options are discussed in **Guide 6**.

> **Ask all the questions. Take a notebook. Advocate for yourself. Assemble your team of people that will lift you up."**

Guide 6
Additional treatments for lower-risk MDS with symptomatic anemia and the *SF3B1* mutation

For people with a serum EPO level of 500 mU/mL or less:	• Imetelstat (preferred) • Epoetin alfa with or without a G-CSF (other recommended) • Darbepoetin alfa with or without a G-CSF (other recommended)	→	If the cancer doesn't respond to treatment or comes back after it went away (relapses), the treatments listed next will be given	→	• See treatment options on page 37 (they are the same in this case) • Ivosidenib, if the *IDH1* gene is mutated (other recommended) • Enasidenib, if the *IDH2* gene is mutated (other recommended)
For people with a serum EPO level more than 500 mU/mL:	• Imetelstat, if not given yet (preferred) • Luspatercept, if not given yet (preferred) • Lenalidomide (other recommended)	→	If the cancer doesn't respond to treatment or comes back after it went away (relapses), the treatments listed next will be given	→	• See treatment options on page 37 (they are the same in this case) • Ivosidenib, if the *IDH1* gene is mutated (other recommended) • Enasidenib, if the *IDH2* gene is mutated (other recommended)

Treatments for lower-risk MDS with symptomatic anemia and no 5q deletion with or without other cytogenetic abnormalities

Treatment for this type of MDS is based on serum EPO levels.

- People with a serum EPO level of 500 mU/mL or less may receive the treatments described in **Guide 7**.
- People with a serum EPO level of more than 500 mU/mL may receive the treatments described on page 37 (treatments are the same in this case).

Guide 7
Treatments for lower-risk MDS with symptomatic anemia and no 5q deletion with or without other cytogenetic abnormalities

For people with a serum EPO level of 500 mU/mL or less:

• Epoetin alfa • Darbepoetin alfa • Luspatercept (preferred for people with a serum EPO level greater than 200 mU/mL) →	**If the cancer responds to treatment:** • Continue treatment, decrease the dose of Epoetin alfa and Darbepoetin alfa **If the cancer doesn't respond to treatment or relapses:** → • Imetelstat (preferred) • Luspatercept, if not given yet (preferred) • Epoetin alfa with or without G-CSF or lenalidomide • Darbepoetin alfa with or without G-CSF or lenalidomide	**If the cancer responds to treatment:** • Continue treatment, decrease the dose of Epoetin alfa and Darbepoetin alfa **If the cancer doesn't respond to treatment or relapses:** • Imetelstat, if not given yet (preferred) • See treatment options on page 37 (they are the same in this case) • Ivosidenib, if the *IDH1* gene is mutated (useful in certain circumstances) • Enasidenib, if the *IDH2* gene is mutated (useful in certain circumstances)

Key points

- Treatment options for lower-risk myelodysplastic syndromes (MDS) are based on many different factors, such as the presence of symptomatic anemia, the genetic and cytogenetic characteristics of the MDS, and your serum erythropoietin (EPO) level. If the cancer doesn't respond to the first treatment given, more options are available.
- People with MDS and clinically relevant thrombocytopenia (low platelet counts) or neutropenia (low counts of neutrophils, a type of white blood cell) can first receive therapy with a clinical trial, azacitidine, decitabine, decitabine and cedazuridine, or immunosuppressive therapy with or without eltrombopag.
- Before people with MDS and symptomatic anemia can be treated, tests are given to learn as much about the anemia as possible.
- Treatment of people with MDS and symptomatic anemia is based on if they have a 5q deletion (known as MDS-5q) or *SF3B1* mutation (known as MDS-SF3B1). It's also based on what their serum EPO level is.
- The first treatment given for people with MDS and symptomatic anemia and the 5q deletion is lenalidomide (preferred). If you have a serum EPO level that's 500 mU/mL or less, epoetin alfa and darbepoetin alfa are other recommended therapy options.
- The first treatments given for people with MDS and symptomatic anemia and the *SF3B1* mutation are luspatercept (preferred) and imetelstat (other recommended, given to people with a serum EPO level greater than 500 mU/mL who can't receive epoetin alfa or darbepoetin alfa).
- The first treatments given for people with MDS, symptomatic anemia, and no 5q deletion with or without other cytogenetic abnormalities depend on what their serum EPO level is.

Questions to ask

- What type of MDS do I have, and what are the best treatments for it?
- How did you pick the treatment plan for me?
- What are my blood counts? What counts are considered high and low?
- What side effects are common with the treatments I might get?
- What services are available to help me with the cost of treatment? Who will connect me with these services and resources?

6
Treating higher-risk MDS

This chapter explains the different treatment options for higher-risk myelodysplastic syndromes (MDS). The treatment you'll receive depends on whether a hematopoietic stem cell transplant is part of your care plan.

The treatments given for higher-risk myelodysplastic syndromes (MDS) depend on if you can have an allogeneic hematopoietic cell transplant. Your care team will look at many factors, including your age, health, and preferences, to figure out if you can get an allogeneic hematopoietic cell transplant.

The sections below describe the treatments for people who might get an allogeneic hematopoietic cell transplant and people who aren't planning to get one.

Treatments for MDS when an allogeneic hematopoietic cell transplant may be given

Guide 8 lists the first treatment options for people with higher-risk MDS who are able to receive an allogeneic hematopoietic cell transplant.

Second treatments

If you haven't received an allogeneic hematopoietic cell transplant yet, these therapies can be given next:

- Allogeneic hematopoietic cell transplant
- Ivosidenib (Tibsovo), if the *IDH1* gene is mutated
- Enasidenib (Idhifa), if the *IDH2* gene is mutated

Guide 8
First treatment options for higher-risk MDS when an allogeneic hematopoietic cell transplant may be given

- Allogeneic hematopoietic cell transplant
- Clinical trial followed by allogeneic hematopoietic cell transplant
- Azacitidine with or without Venetoclax
- Decitabine with or without Venetoclax
- Decitabine and cedazuridine with or without Venetoclax
- High-intensity chemotherapy

If the cancer doesn't respond to treatment or relapses after the transplant

There are more treatment options if the cancer doesn't respond to treatment or comes back after an allogeneic hematopoietic cell transplant. Treatments that may be given are:

- Another allogeneic hematopoietic cell transplant or an infusion of lymphocytes (a type of white blood cell) from a donor
- Clinical trial
- Azacitidine (Vidaza)
- Decitabine
- Decitabine and cedazuridine (Inqovi)

After this treatment is given, your care team will check on you again. If the cancer is responding to treatment, you'll continue to receive the same treatment. If the cancer isn't responding or relapses, a clinical trial or supportive care may be offered.

Higher-risk MDS includes Revised International Prognostic Scoring System (IPSS-R) intermediate-risk, high-risk, and very high-risk groups.

Treatments for MDS when an allogeneic hematopoietic cell transplant isn't planned

If an allogeneic hematopoietic cell transplant isn't the right treatment for you, many other treatments are available. **Guide 9** describes these options.

If one is available, a clinical trial is another option for people who have received ivosidenib.

Guide 9
Treatments for higher-risk MDS when an allogeneic hematopoietic cell transplant isn't planned

- Azacitidine (preferred)
- Decitabine (preferred)
- Decitabine and cedazuridine (preferred)
- Clinical trial
- Azacitidine, decitabine, or decitabine and cedazuridine plus Venetoclax (useful in certain circumstances)

→

Additional treatments given if the cancer doesn't respond to treatment or relapses:

- Ivosidenib, if the *IDH1* gene is mutated and it hasn't been given yet
- Enasidenib, if the *IDH2* gene is mutated
- Clinical trial
- Azacitidine, decitabine, or decitabine and cedazuridine plus Venetoclax, if it hasn't been given yet

Key points

- Treatments are different for people with higher-risk myelodysplastic syndromes (MDS) who are eligible to receive an allogeneic hematopoietic cell transplant and those who are not.
- The first treatment options for people with higher-risk MDS who are eligible to receive an allogeneic hematopoietic cell transplant are an allogeneic hematopoietic cell transplant; a clinical trial followed by the transplant; azacitidine, decitabine, or decitabine and cedazuridine with or without venetoclax; and high-intensity chemotherapy.
- The first treatment options for people with higher-risk MDS who are not eligible to receive an allogeneic hematopoietic cell transplant are azacitidine (preferred); decitabine (preferred); decitabine and cedazuridine (preferred); a clinical trial (if available); and azacitidine, decitabine, or decitabine and cedazuridine with or without venetoclax (useful in certain circumstances).
- Other treatment options are available if the cancer doesn't respond to treatment with the first therapy or comes back after treatment (relapses).

Questions to ask

- What treatment would you recommend for me and why?
- Is an allogeneic hematopoietic cell transplant a treatment option for me?
- Can you tell me about the process of an allogeneic hematopoietic cell transplant? Will I have to stay in the hospital after the procedure?
- What side effects are common with the treatments I might get?
- What services are available to help me with the cost of treatment? Who will connect me with these services and resources?

We want your feedback!

Our goal is to provide helpful and easy-to-understand information on cancer. Take our survey to let us know what we got right and what we could do better.
NCCN.org/patients/feedback

7

MDS/MPN overlap syndromes

In uncommon cases, blood cancer can have features of myelodysplastic syndromes (MDS) and myeloproliferative neoplasms (MPN). MDS/MPN overlap syndromes are when the cancer has characteristics of both MDS and MPN. This chapter explains the different overlap syndromes and how they're treated.

What's the difference between MDS and MPN, and what's MDS/MPN overlap?

Myelodysplastic syndromes (MDS) are a group of diseases where the bone marrow doesn't make enough healthy mature blood cells (red blood cells, white blood cells, and/or platelets).

Myeloproliferative neoplasms (MPN) are a group of diseases where the bone marrow makes too many of 1 or more types of blood cells (red blood cells, white blood cells, and/or platelets).

Although it's uncommon, MDS can sometimes overlap with MPN. When this happens, blood cancer has features of both MDS and MPN.

Types of MDS/MPN

The following are types of MDS/MPN according to the 2022 classification system from the World Health Organization (WHO):

- Chronic myelomonocytic leukemia (CMML)
- MDS/MPN and neutrophilia
- MDS/MPN with an *SF3B1* mutation and thrombocytosis
- MDS/MPN not otherwise specified (also called MDS/MPN NOS)
- MPN

CMML

CMML is a disease where the bone marrow makes too many monocytes (a type of white blood cell). Monocytes and sometimes blasts then crowd out and overwhelm the other cells in the bone marrow. As a result, there are not enough red blood cells, platelets, and healthy white blood cells.

The WHO categorizes CMML into 2 subtypes (CMML-1 and CMML-2) based on the number of blasts found in the bone marrow.

MDS/MPN and neutrophilia

MDS/MPN and neutrophilia is a disease where the bone marrow makes too many neutrophils (a type of white blood cell). Neutrophils and sometimes blasts then crowd out and overwhelm the other cells in the bone marrow, so there aren't enough red blood cells, platelets, and healthy white blood cells.

MDS/MPN with an *SF3B1* mutation and thrombocytosis

MDS/MPN with an *SF3B1* mutation and thrombocytosis is a disease where there's an *SF3B1* mutation, anemia (low red blood cell counts), thrombocytosis (high platelet counts), and ring sideroblasts (immature red blood cells with too much iron).

MDS/MPN not otherwise specified

This subtype of MDS/MPN includes blood cancer that has features of MDS and MPN but doesn't fit into the other subtype categories.

MPN

To learn more about MPN specifically, see *NCCN Guidelines for Patients: Myeloproliferative Neoplasms*, available at NCCN.org/patientguidelines and on the NCCN Patient Guides for Cancer app.

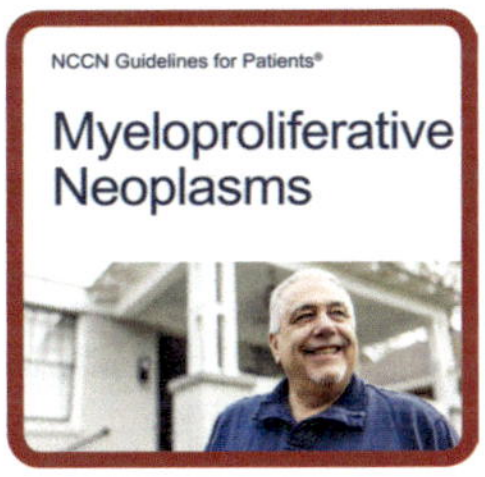

Treatment for MDS/MPN

Treatment options for MDS/MPN overlap syndromes are based on what subtype of MDS/MPN you have and what blood cell abnormalities are the most common. There are different options, such as an allogeneic hematopoietic cell transplant (also called a bone marrow or stem cell transplant) and a type of therapy called hypomethylating agents.

For information on the specific subtypes of MDS/MPN and their treatment options, see **Guide 10**.

Guide 10
Treatments for MDS/MPN overlap syndromes

Subtype	Treatment
Chronic myelomonocytic leukemia (CMML)	For CMML-1: Consider chemotherapy or hydroxyurea For CMML-2: Chemotherapy with or without venetoclax and/or allogeneic hematopoietic cell transplant
MDS/MPN and neutrophilia	Consider chemotherapy and/or ruxolitinib and/or allogeneic hematopoietic cell transplant
MDS/MPN with *SF3B1* mutation and thrombocytosis	Consider chemotherapy and/or lenalidomide or consider luspatercept
MDS/MPN, not otherwise specified (NOS)	Consider chemotherapy and/or allogeneic hematopoietic cell transplant
MPN	Allogeneic hematopoietic cell transplant

Key points

- Although it's uncommon, myelodysplastic syndromes (MDS) can sometimes overlap with myeloproliferative neoplasms (MPN). When this happens, blood cancer has features of both MDS and MPN.
- MDS is a group of diseases in which bone marrow does not make enough healthy mature blood cells (red blood cells, white blood cells, and/or platelets). In MPN, the body makes too many of 1 or more types of blood cells.
- Treatment options for MDS/MPN overlap syndromes are based on the subtype of MDS/MPN and what blood cell abnormalities are the most common.
- The subtypes of MDS/MPN according to the 2022 classification system from the World Health Organization (WHO) are chronic myelomonocytic leukemia (CMML), MDS/MPN and neutrophilia, MDS/MPN with an *SF3B1* mutation and thrombocytosis, MDS/MPN not otherwise specified (also called MDS/MPN NOS), and MPN.
- Treatment options can include an allogeneic hematopoietic cell transplant, hypomethylating agents, and other drugs.

Questions to ask

- What type of MDS/MPN do I have?
- What treatments are options for me? What's it like getting these treatments? Will I need to stay in the hospital?
- What services are available to help me with the cost of treatment? Who will connect me with these services and resources?
- What side effects are common with the treatments I might get?
- Who do I call if I have side effects when the doctor's office is closed?

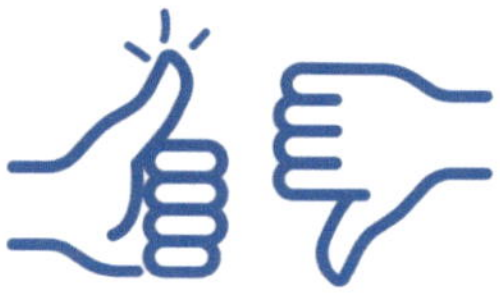

Let us know what you think!

Please take a moment to complete an online survey about the NCCN Guidelines for Patients.
NCCN.org/patients/response

8
Other resources

Want to learn more? Here's how you can get additional help.

What else to know

This guide helps you know your options so you can make informed decisions and improve your cancer care. But it's not the only resource that you have.

Ask for as much information and help as you need. Many people are interested in learning more about:

- Blood cancer and the type of MDS they have
- If they need to go to a specialized care center to get treatment for MDS
- How hypomethylating agents are different from typical chemotherapy
- What an allogeneic hematopoietic cell transplant is like and how the procedure works
- How to manage the side effects of low blood cell counts

What else to do

Your health care center can help you with next steps. It often has on-site resources to help meet your needs and find answers to your questions. Health care centers can also inform you of resources in your community.

In addition to help from your providers, the resources listed in the next section provide support for many people like yourself.

Where to get help

Look through the list below and visit the provided websites to learn more about these organizations.

Blood Cancer United
bloodcancerunited.org

BMT InfoNet
bmtinfonet.org

CancerCare
cancercare.org

Healthtree Foundation
healthtree.org

Imerman Angels
imermanangels.org

Leukemia Research Foundation
leukemiarf.org

MDS Foundation
MDS-foundation.org

National Bone Marrow Transplant Link (nbmtLINK)
nbmtlink.org

NMDP
nmdp.org/one-on-one

PAN Foundation
panfoundation.org

TargetCancer Foundation
targetcancer.org

Triage Cancer
triagecancer.org

"

Setting a goal, giving myself something positive to do and focusing on the training for it mentally was very crucial for my recovery, I believe."

Questions to ask

- If I live far from specialized MDS hospitals and care centers, how can I make sure I'm getting the best treatment?
- What resources are available to help me pay for care, get transportation to care, find childcare while I'm getting care, and more?
- What side effects should I look out for during treatment, and what should I do if I experience them?
- What side effects does someone with my type of MDS usually experience? What helps them feel better?
- How does the hematopoietic cell transplant process work? Can my family do a test to see if they're a match to donate stem cells to me?

Words to know

acute myeloid leukemia (AML)
A fast-growing cancer in which the bone marrow makes abnormal and immature white blood cells called blasts. MDS can sometimes turn into AML.

allogeneic hematopoietic cell transplant
A treatment that uses healthy hematopoietic (blood-forming) cells from another person (donor) to regrow your bone marrow after you receive chemotherapy and/or radiation therapy to kill cancer cells.

anemia
Having low red blood cell counts.

blast cell
An immature blood cell. Normal bone marrow contains some healthy blasts, which make other normal blood cells (red blood cells, white blood cells, platelets). In MDS, the number of blasts can increase. These extra blasts are abnormal and cannot make normal blood cells. The abnormal blasts in MDS can crowd out the bone marrow and stop normal cells from growing.

blood stem cell
An immature blood-forming cell from which other types of blood cells are made. Also called a hematopoietic stem cell.

bone marrow
The soft, spongy tissue in the center of most bones where blood cells are made.

bone marrow aspiration and biopsy
The removal of a small amount of liquid and solid part of the bone marrow. This is done to diagnose MDS and figure out what type of MDS you have.

chemotherapy
Treatment that kills cancer cells throughout the body.

clinical trial
A type of medical research study that tests new ways of fighting cancer in people.

complete blood count
A test that measures the number of red blood cells, white blood cells, and platelets in your blood.

cytogenetic testing
A test that uses samples of your tissue, blood, or bone marrow to look for changes and abnormalities in chromosomes.

cytopenia
A condition where the counts of certain types of blood cells are low. Anemia, leukopenia, neutropenia, and thrombocytopenia are all types of cytopenias.

diagnosis
The identification of an illness based on tests.

donor
A person who gives their organs, tissues, or stem cells to another person.

erythropoiesis-stimulating agents (ESAs)
Drugs that kick-start the bone marrow to make more red blood cells.

erythropoietin (EPO)
A hormone in the body that tells (stimulates) the bone marrow to make more red blood cells. Erythropoietin is produced by the kidneys.

fatigue
Severe tiredness, despite getting enough sleep, that limits one's ability to function.

flow cytometry
A lab test that uses a blood, tissue, or bone marrow sample to count, identify, sort, and classify cells. This test is used to help diagnose MDS.

fluorescence in situ hybridization (FISH)
A test that detects specific common chromosome changes known to affect people with MDS.

genetic testing
Tests that look for mutations in genes (sequences of DNA).

granulocyte colony-stimulating factor (G-CSF)
A drug that's given to help increase white blood cell counts.

human leukocyte antigen (HLA) typing
A test to determine which donor is the best match for a hemopoietic cell transplant.

immune system
The body's natural defense against infection and disease.

immunosuppressive therapy (IST)
Drugs that weaken the body's immune system. This type of therapy is sometimes given to prevent the immune system from attacking healthy cells.

intravenous (IV)
An injection into a vein.

karyotype
A picture of all of someone's chromosomes.

lactate dehydrogenase (LDH)
A protein found in almost all cells. This protein is released into the blood when cells die.

leukopenia
Having low white blood cell counts.

medical history
A complete report of your health.

molecular testing
A type of genetic testing that examines DNA. Polymerase chain reaction (PCR) and next-generation sequencing (NGS) are examples of molecular tests.

mutation
A change in the structure of a gene. Mutations are often considered abnormal, but some mutations are harmless.

MDS/MPN overlap syndromes
When a blood cancer has characteristics of both MDS and MPN.

myelodysplastic syndromes (MDS)
A group of diseases where the bone marrow doesn't make enough healthy, mature blood cells (red blood cells, white blood cells, and/or platelets). MDS is a type of blood cancer.

myeloproliferative neoplasms (MPN)
A group of diseases where the bone marrow makes too many blood cells (red blood cells, white blood cells, and/or platelets). MPN is a type of blood cancer.

next-generation sequencing
A test that checks the sequence (order) of genes to look for mutations and changes.

neutropenia
A type of leukopenia where there are low counts of a type of white blood cell called neutrophils. Neutrophils are responsible for fighting infections.

platelet
A type of blood cell that helps control bleeding.

polymerase chain reaction (PCR)
A test that creates many copies of a specific gene so DNA can be better examined.

prognosis
The likely or expected course and outcome of a disease.

red blood cell
A type of blood cell that carries oxygen from the lungs to the rest of the body.

relapse
The return or worsening of cancer after a period of improvement.

Revised International Prognostic Scoring System (IPSS-R)
A system that health care providers use to rate the severity of MDS and classify it into groups based on the likely outcome (prognosis). It places people with MDS into 1 of the following 5 groups: very low risk, low risk, intermediate risk, high risk, or very high risk.

ring sideroblasts
Immature red blood cells that have too much iron and show up as a circle (ring) around the center of the cells.

risk group
The classification of MDS based on severity and the chance (risk) that it will progress to AML.

side effect
An unhealthy or unpleasant physical or emotional condition caused by treatment.

subtype
Smaller groups that a type of cancer is divided into based on certain features of the cancer cells.

supportive care
Supportive care prevents or manages the symptoms of cancer and the side effects of cancer treatment. It also addresses mental, social, emotional, and spiritual concerns.

symptom
Usually unpleasant feelings that can be a sign of a disease or condition.

systemic therapy
Treatment that works throughout the entire body. It can be in form of pills or injections. Chemotherapy is a type of systemic therapy.

targeted therapy
Treatment that targets specific features of cancer cells.

thrombocytopenia
Having low platelet counts.

transfusion
A slow infusion of red blood cells or platelets into a vein.

white blood cell
A type of blood cell that helps fight infections in the body. There are different types of white blood cells (neutrophils, lymphocytes, monocytes, eosinophils, and basophils).

NCCN Contributors

This patient guide is based on the NCCN Clinical Practice Guidelines in Oncology (NCCN Guidelines®) for Myelodysplastic Syndromes, Version 3.2026. It was adapted, reviewed, and published with help from the following people:

Dorothy A. Shead, MS
Senior Director
Patient Information Operations

Megan Hollasch
Medical Writer

Lisa Diehl
Production Layout Artist

The NCCN Clinical Practice Guidelines in Oncology (NCCN Guidelines®) for Myelodysplastic Syndromes, Version 3.2026, were developed by the following NCCN Panel Members:

*Peter L. Greenberg, MD/Chair
Stanford Cancer Institute

Richard M. Stone, MD/Vice Chair
Dana-Farber/Brigham and Women's Cancer Center

Yasmin Abaza, MD
Robert H. Lurie Comprehensive Cancer Center of Northwestern University

Aref Al-Kali, MD
Mayo Clinic Comprehensive Cancer Center

Sarah Anand, MD
University of Michigan Rogel Cancer Center

Kimo Bachiashvili, MD
O'Neal Comprehensive Cancer Center at UAB

Brian Ball, MD, MS
City of Hope National Medical Center

John M. Bennett, MD
University of Rochester

*Krist Biakanja III
Patient Advocate

Uma Borate, MD, MSc
The Ohio State University Comprehensive Cancer Center - James Cancer Hospital and Solove Research Institute

Andrew M. Brunner, MD
Mass General Cancer Center

Rebecca Bystrom, MD
Duke Cancer Institute

Wanxing Chai-Ho, MD
UCLA Jonsson Comprehensive Cancer Center

Kelly Chien, MD
The University of Texas MD Anderson Cancer Center

Amy E. DeZern, MD, MHS
Johns Hopkins Kimmel Cancer Center

Karin Gaensler, MD
UCSF Helen Diller Family Comprehensive Cancer Center

Zhubin Gahvari, MD
University of Wisconsin Carbone Cancer Center

Elizabeth A. Griffiths, MD
Roswell Park Comprehensive Cancer Center

Tamanna Haque, MD
Memorial Sloan Kettering Cancer Center

Meagan Jacoby, MD, PhD
Siteman Cancer Center at Barnes-Jewish Hospital and Washington University School of Medicine

Brian A. Jonas, MD, PhD
UC Davis Comprehensive Cancer Center

Sioban Keel, MD
Fred Hutchinson Cancer Center

Rashmi Khanal, MD
Fox Chase Cancer Center

Ashwin Kishtagari, MD
Vanderbilt-Ingram Cancer Center

Yazan Madanat, MD
UT Southwestern Simmons Comprehensive Cancer Center

Lori J. Maness, MD
Fred & Pamela Buffett Cancer Center

Shannon McCurdy, MD
Abramson Cancer Center at the University of Pennsylvania

Christine McMahon, MD
University of Colorado Cancer Center

Olatoyosi Odenike, MD
The UChicago Medicine Comprehensive Cancer Center

Afaf Osman, MD
Huntsman Cancer Institute at the University of Utah

Vishnu V. Reddy, MD
O'Neal Comprehensive Cancer Center at UAB

David A. Sallman, MD
Moffitt Cancer Center

*Hamid Sayar, MD, MSc
Indiana University Melvin and Bren Simon Comprehensive Cancer Center

Abhay Singh, MD, MPH
Case Comprehensive Cancer Center/ University Hospitals Seidman Cancer Center and Cleveland Clinic Taussig Cancer Institute

*Maximilian Stahl, MD
Yale Cancer Center/Smilow Cancer Hospital

Tiffany Tanaka, MD
UC San Diego Moores Cancer Center

Swapna Thota, MD
St. Jude Children's Research Hospital/ The University of Tennessee Health Science Center

NCCN

Cindy Hochstetler, PhD
Oncology Scientist/Senior Medical Writer

Emily Kovach
Guidelines Layout Specialist

Jamie Nguyen, PharmD
Associate Scientist/Medical Writer

*Reviewed this patient guide. For disclosures, visit NCCN.org/disclosures.

NCCN Cancer Centers

For contact information, visit NCCN.org/cancercenters.

Abramson Cancer Center
at the University of Pennsylvania
Philadelphia, Pennsylvania

Case Comprehensive Cancer Center/
University Hospitals Seidman Cancer Center and
Cleveland Clinic Taussig Cancer Institute
Cleveland, Ohio

City of Hope National Medical Center
Duarte, California

Dana-Farber/Brigham and Women's Cancer Center |
Mass General Cancer Center
Boston, Massachusetts

Duke Cancer Institute
Durham, North Carolina

Fox Chase Cancer Center
Philadelphia, Pennsylvania

Fred & Pamela Buffett Cancer Center
Omaha, Nebraska

Fred Hutchinson Cancer Center
Seattle, Washington

Huntsman Cancer Institute at the University of Utah
Salt Lake City, Utah

Indiana University Melvin and Bren Simon
Comprehensive Cancer Center
Indianapolis, Indiana

Johns Hopkins Kimmel Cancer Center
Baltimore, Maryland

Mayo Clinic Comprehensive Cancer Center
Phoenix/Scottsdale, Arizona
Jacksonville, Florida
Rochester, Minnesota

Memorial Sloan Kettering Cancer Center
New York, New York

Moffitt Cancer Center
Tampa, Florida

O'Neal Comprehensive Cancer Center at UAB
Birmingham, Alabama

Robert H. Lurie Comprehensive Cancer Center
of Northwestern University
Chicago, Illinois

Roswell Park Comprehensive Cancer Center
Buffalo, New York

Siteman Cancer Center at Barnes-Jewish Hospital
and Washington University School of Medicine
St. Louis, Missouri

St. Jude Children's Research Hospital/
The University of Tennessee Health Science Center
Memphis, Tennessee

Stanford Cancer Institute
Stanford, California

The Ohio State University Comprehensive Cancer Center -
James Cancer Hospital and Solove Research Institute
Columbus, Ohio

The UChicago Medicine Comprehensive Cancer Center
Chicago, Illinois

The University of Texas MD Anderson Cancer Center
Houston, Texas

UC Davis Comprehensive Cancer Center
Sacramento, California

UC San Diego Moores Cancer Center
La Jolla, California

UCLA Jonsson Comprehensive Cancer Center
Los Angeles, California

UCSF Helen Diller Family Comprehensive Cancer Center
San Francisco, California

University of Colorado Cancer Center
Aurora, Colorado

University of Michigan Rogel Cancer Center
Ann Arbor, Michigan

University of Wisconsin Carbone Cancer Center
Madison, Wisconsin

UT Southwestern Simmons
Comprehensive Cancer Center
Dallas, Texas

Vanderbilt-Ingram Cancer Center
Nashville, Tennessee

Yale Cancer Center/Smilow Cancer Hospital
New Haven, Connecticut

Index

Made in the USA
Monee, IL
05 November 2026

67987968R00036